MEG AND MATTHEW LEAL

It's the Way God Made Me

A memoir of a little boy and his family's journey with severe food allergies

First edition

This book was professionally typeset on Reedsy.
Find out more at reedsy.com

To Michael, an amazing husband and father of my beautiful son,
for our wonderful life.
To Matthew, my artistic partner, favorite little boy
and the joy of my life.
– Meg
To all my friends who keep me safe and alive!
And to my cat, Murray.
– Matthew

Foreword

When Matthew was 6, we wrote and illustrated a book called *The Adventures of Elemental P.* We wrote this book when Matthew was in kindergarten and it contains all the clever ideas and sayings that kids learn when they are first learning to read and write numbers. This book is different.

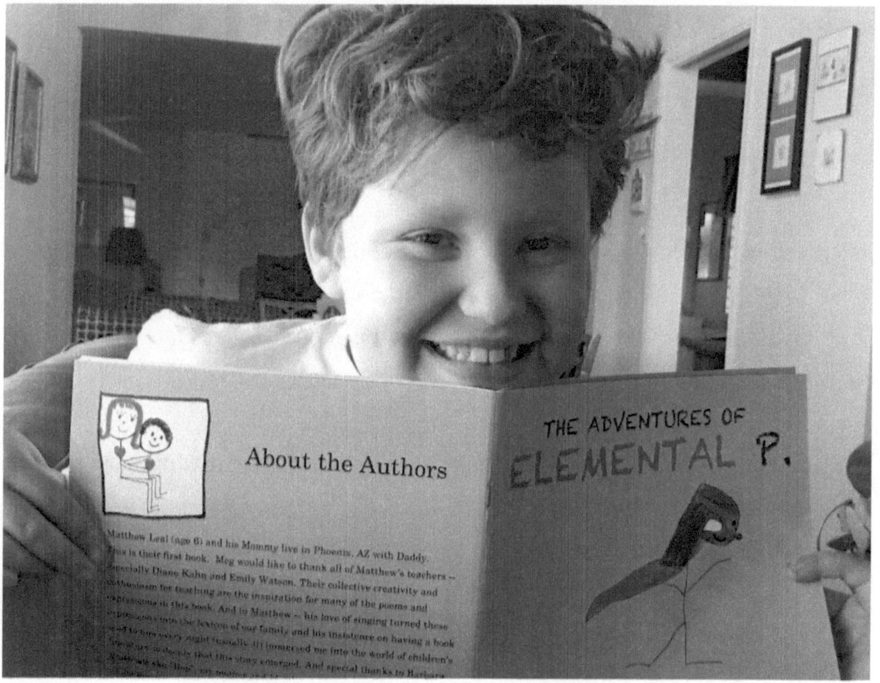

Matthew and our first book.

The Adventures of Elemental P is a learning book. We read it and give it to kids in kindergarten and first grade and they really like it and think it is funny.

This is the story of Matthew and his severe food allergies. He is allergic to peanuts AND tree nuts. Here is a list of the tree nuts Matthew is allergic to:

Almond

Brazil nut

Beechnut

Chestnut

Coconut

Macadamia nut

Pecan

Pine nut

Pistachio

Cashew

Hazelnut

Walnut

Phew! It's a lot.

I don't think people will want to read a book about my food allergies. But I agreed to write it because we could have people read about it instead of having to explain it all the time, especially when I go someplace new. Sometimes I feel weird talking about this to adults I barely know.

I wanted to write this book for different reasons. Not just to share our journey with those who may be on a similar one, but so that maybe people will begin to better understand food allergies. I hope it might save a life- maybe even Matthew's. And I hope it showcases Matthew's amazing spirit and that sometimes a bad thing in your life can turn into something really good.

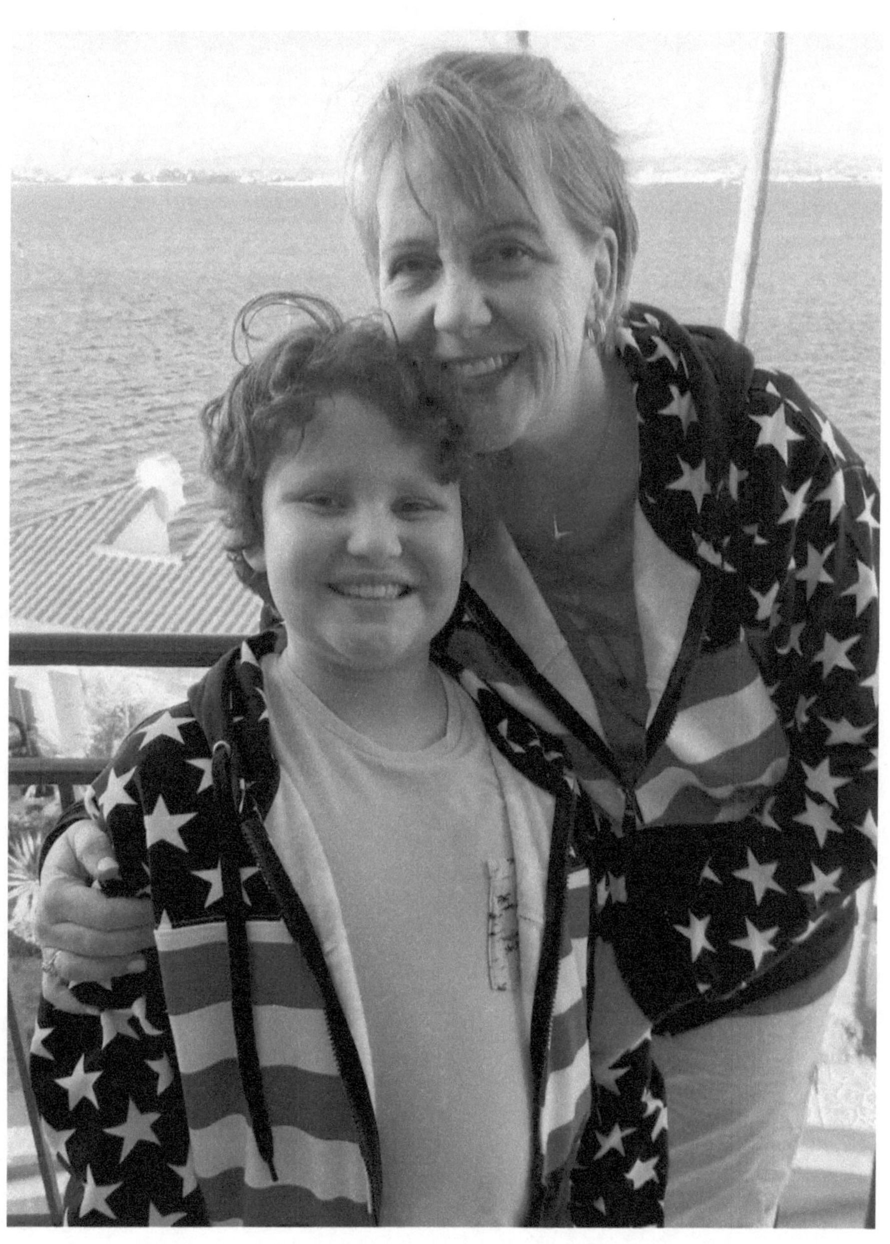

The authors, 2019.

1

"How Did You Find Out?"

No one really asks me this question. But if they do, I just tell them it is a long story and to ask Mommy. I don't remember. I was just a baby. All I know is I have never been able to eat nuts.

This is always the first question people ask me when they learn about his allergy. When he was 22 months old, he ate part of a muffin that had nuts on it. Even though I took the nuts from it, after a few minutes Matthew started to cough. That barky, hacky cough that freaks us allergy moms out. But I didn't know he was allergic, so it didn't upset me at the time. I thought maybe he was getting a cold. (Ignorance is bliss!) Then I spotted some hives on him. His Godmother, an experienced mom and teacher, suggested I give him an antihistamine, even though he was under two. It worked. Problem solved.

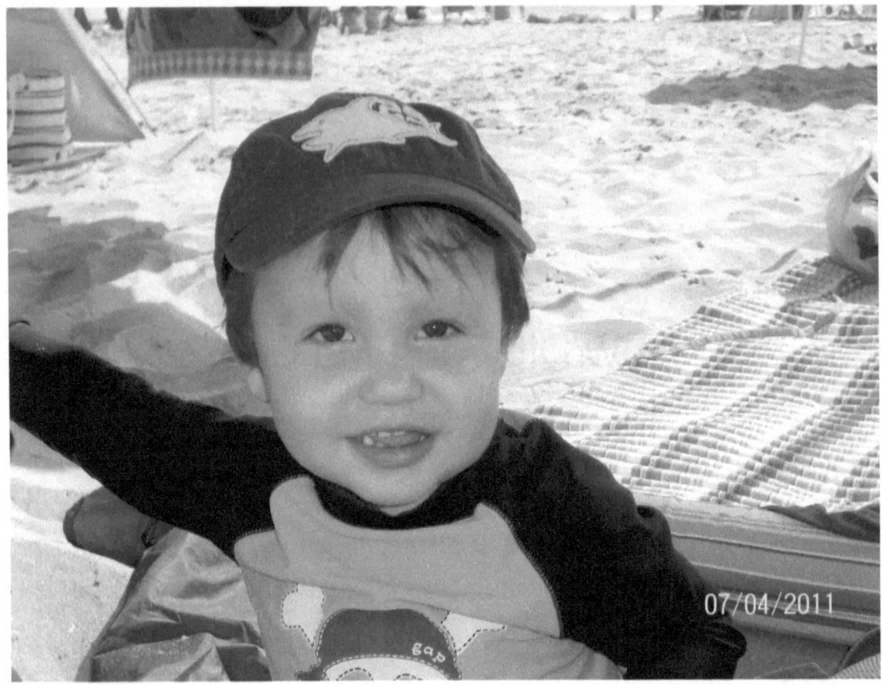

Matthew, 22 months.

Other mom friends, after hearing this story, suggested I get him allergy tested. So did his pediatrician. We went in for the skin tests and he was allergic - but only to cashews and hazelnuts. The muffin I gave him was banana walnut. The doctor said his reaction was probably due to cross contamination and told us to avoid all nuts. They gave us an epinephrine-autoinjector ("epi-pen") and told us to carry it and an antihistamine. He was still in diapers, so it was no big deal to have it in his diaper bag.

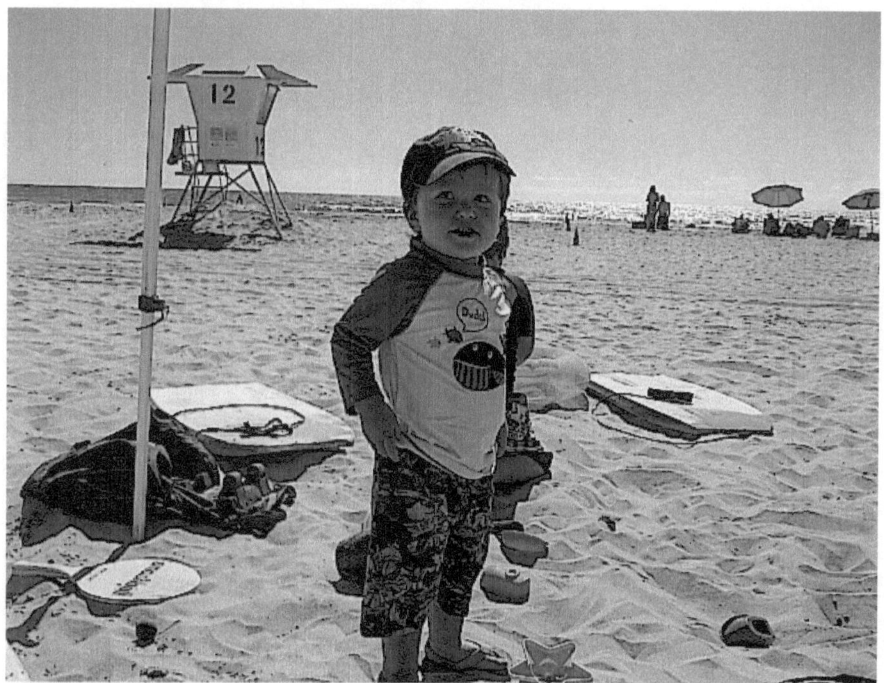

Matthew, age 22 months, he had his first allergic reaction while we were on vacation at the beach.

By now, I had started to hear of other kids with food allergies – eggs, dairy, wheat - and I felt lucky. We only had to worry about nuts.

And originally, he wasn't allergic to peanuts. Which made our lives a lot easier. But there were a few occasions where he reported feeling itchy when someone was eating peanut butter and that was followed by some intestinal distress, so we had him tested when he was seven– and that was when we added peanuts to the list.

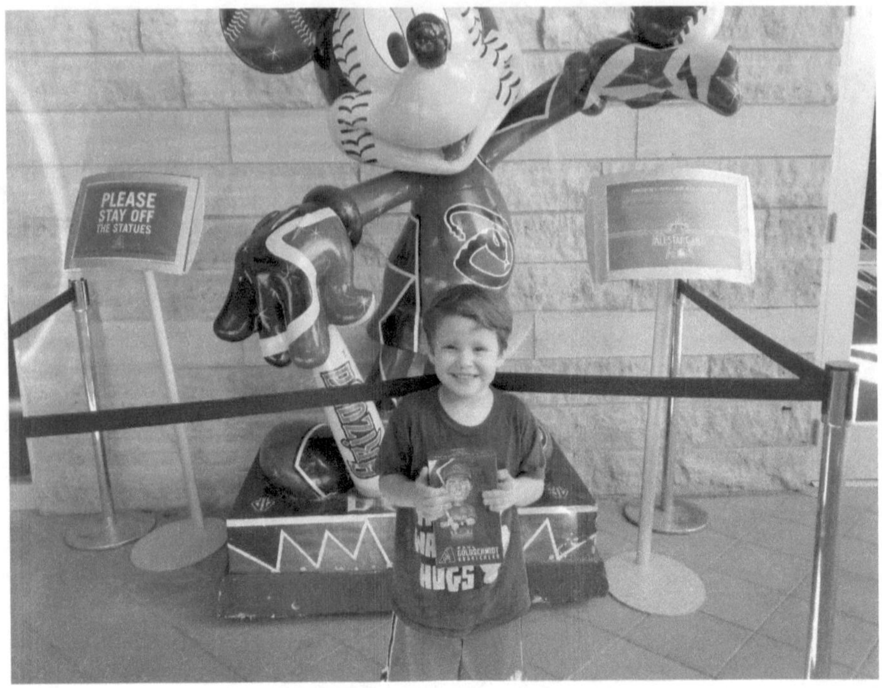

Matthew, age 6, at his first and likely only baseball game, before he was allergic to peanuts.

Over time, like a lot of "allergy " kids we have learned that Matthew is allergic to a few other things. Latex, trees, grass and dogs are the big ones. But he is only mildly allergic to those things and they are easily controlled though avoidance and antihistamines. Luckiest of all, he does not have asthma OR eczema - something almost all allergy kids suffer from. And ironically he is not allergic to cats.

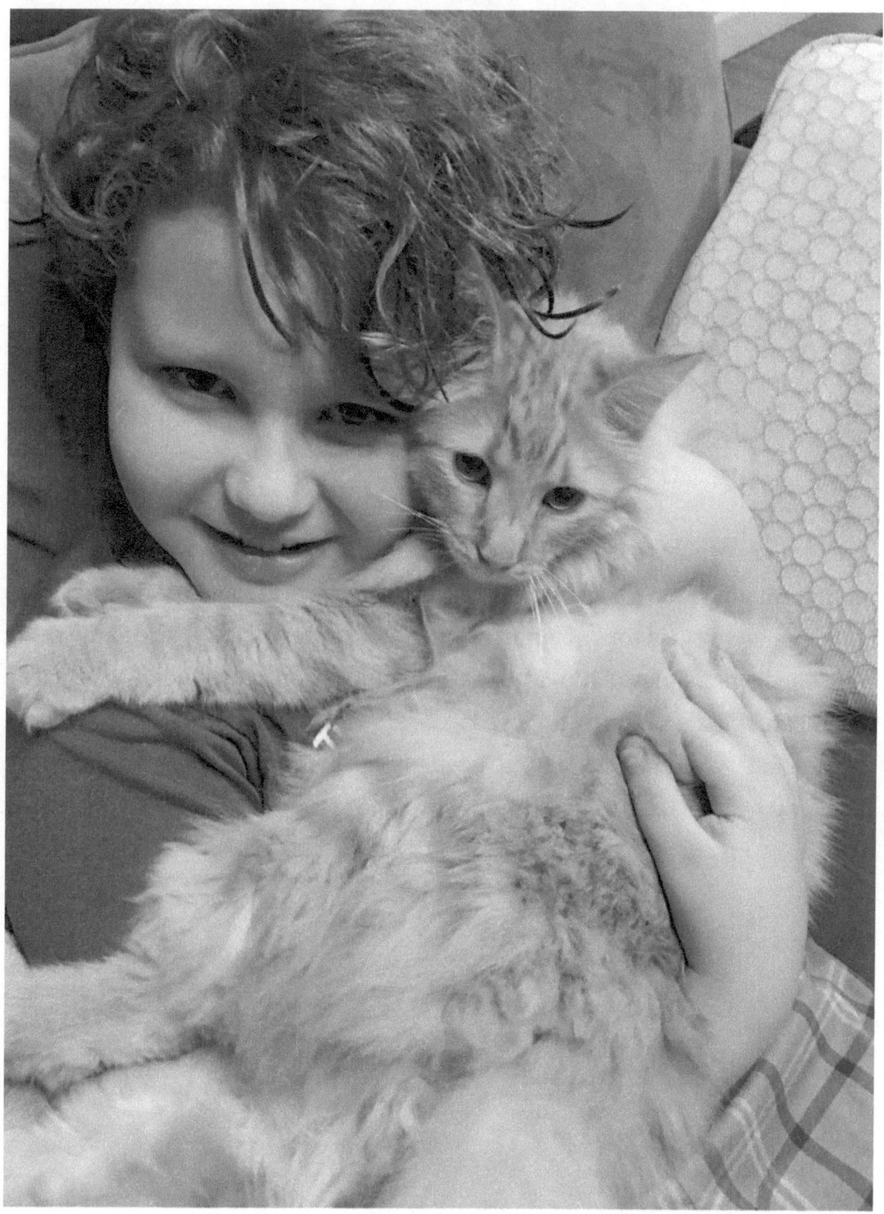

Matthew and his beloved cat, Murray.

2

"He's Anaphylactic!"

The first year that we learned of Matthew's allergies - even though we never let him eat any nuts – he had a few reactions. His eyes swelled and he began to cough when my Dad touched him after eating some cashews. The same thing happened when I kissed him after eating some pecan cake, and he was asleep when I ate it and not even supposed to be allergic to pecans! Aside from those incidents, it was relatively easy to keep his world nut free. Especially because his world was small since he was only two and stayed at home with his Nanny.

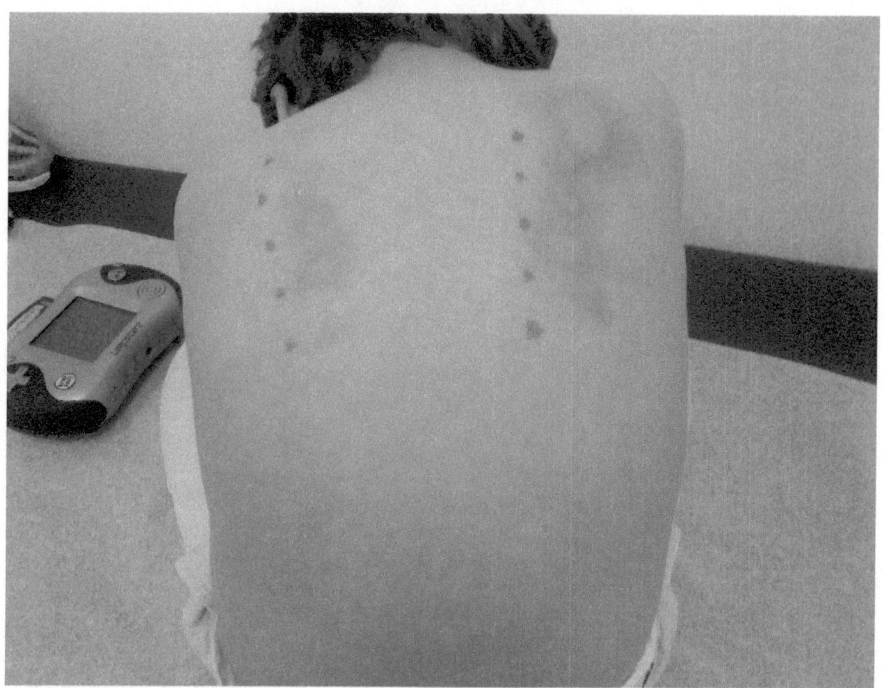

Matthew's first allergy test. He was only allergic to hazelnuts and cashews.

When we went for his next allergy test at age three, he reacted strongly to every single nut including coconut. The hives on his back were huge and his lips started to swell. The Doctor stopped the test halfway through and gave him an antihistamine and made us stay at the office for 45 minutes until the reaction subsided. His allergies were off the charts and now I knew why he had those two reactions after just being touched by someone who had eaten nuts.

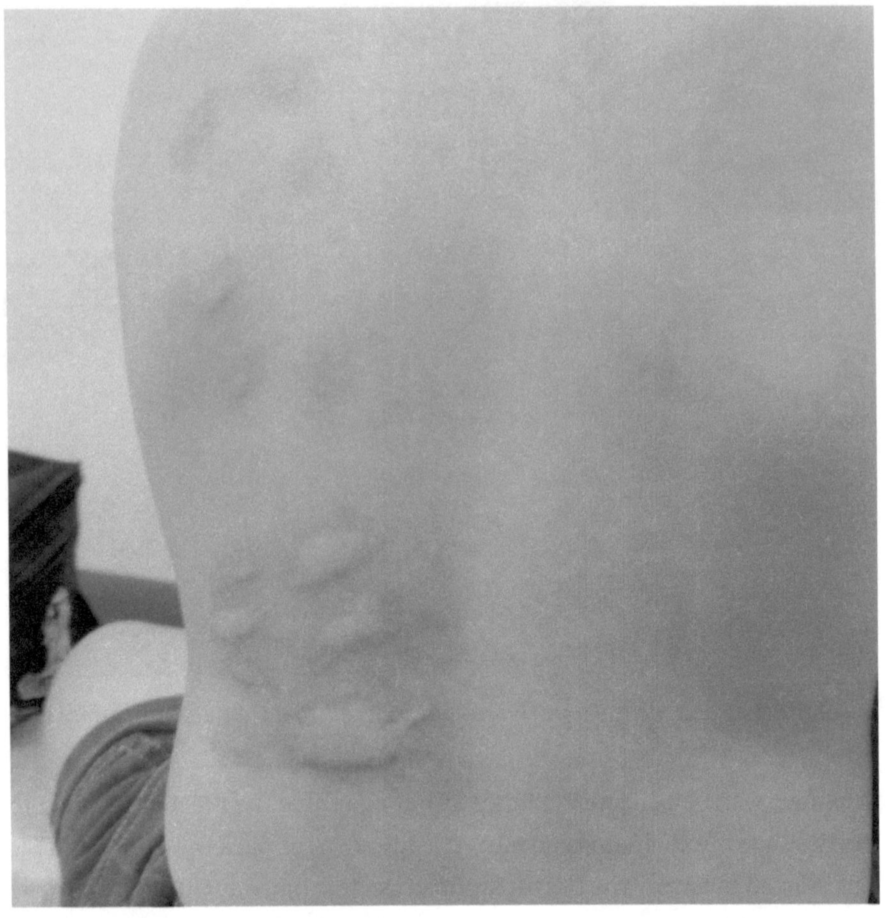

2013 allergy test. They stopped the test because he reacted so strongly.

His allergy was deadly. And he was particularly at risk since it could be caused by just touching him. At three-years-old, he touched everything, and everyone touched him. Nuts became the equivalent of a loaded gun to me. And I was scared.

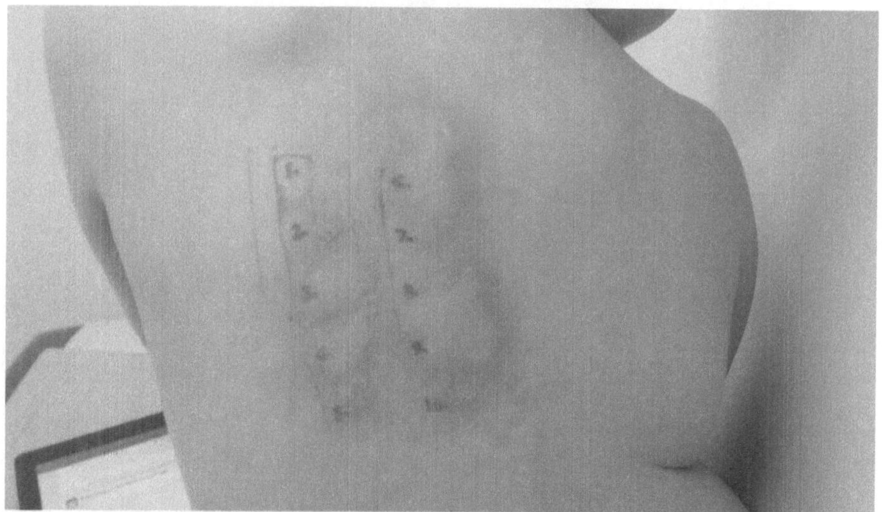

2015 test. Reaction is much worse.

Because the skin tests were painful to Matthew it was easy to convince him to stay away from nuts. We never let him have any food unless we handed it to him. He learned not to eat anything without asking about nuts.

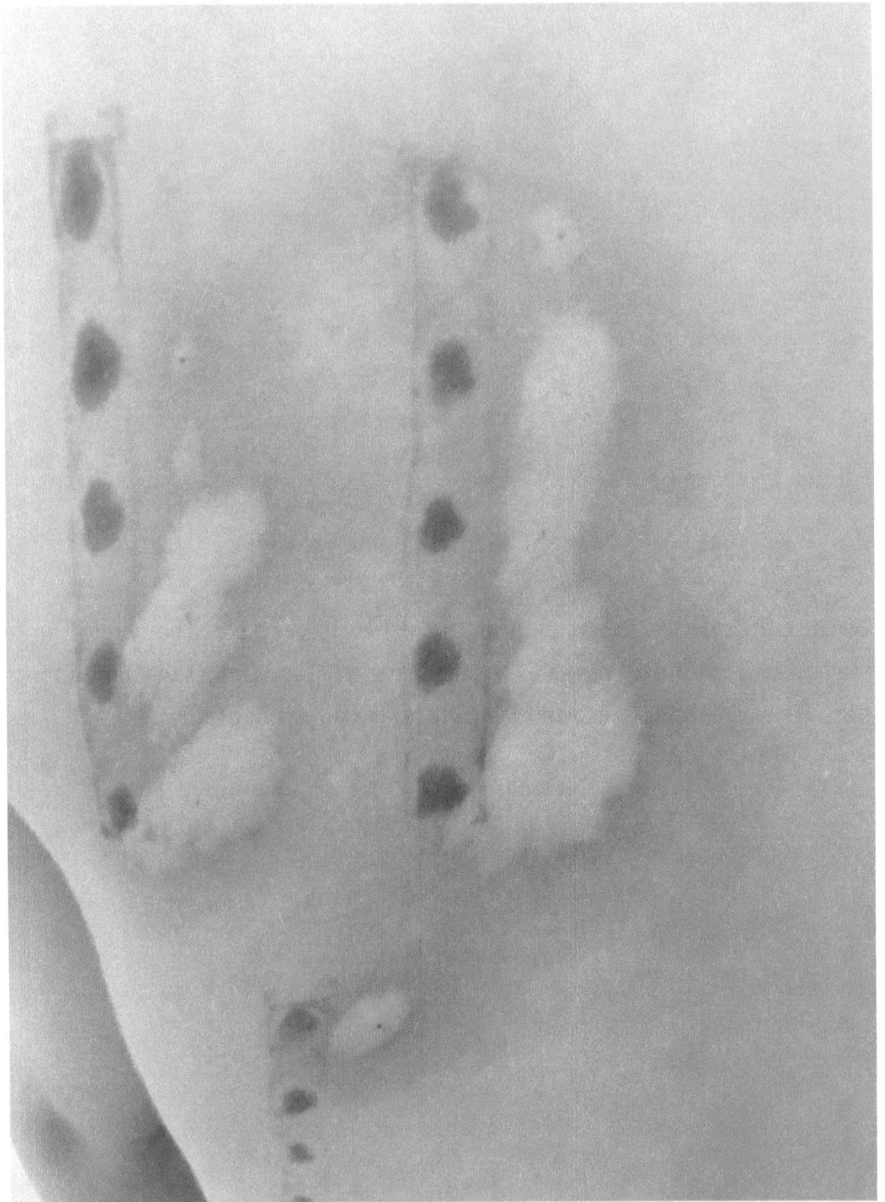

2016 test. After this, they stopped doing skin tests for fear it would send him into anaphylaxis.

A lot of food tastes disgusting to me. Like if there are too many flavors. I can always tell if something is made differently from the way I had it last time. It took a while *to get my mommy and daddy to understand that too many flavors mixed together is disgusting to me. Sometimes they got mad at me when I said I wouldn't eat something – like when Mommy made lasagna. I like everything in it and I like to help make it, but I won't eat it.*

3

"It's Sneaky."

Because Matthew's allergies are so severe, we must be on the lookout for nuts in everything. And his allergy seems to have coincided with the rise in popularity of nuts as a healthy food choice and a substitute for people with different food allergies. Almond flour for gluten-free, almond milk for dairy free, coconut oil as a healthy fat, and coconut water as a healthy substitute for juice boxes – it is everywhere! As a result of this we read every food label every time he eats something. Coconut oil in particular seems to be in everything from ice cream sandwiches to fruit gummies to popcorn. And since the oils are not regulated as to whether they contain nut proteins or just the oil, we must avoid them all.

Sometimes I forget to be careful. One time, I ate some popcorn that I had eaten before. When Mommy saw me eating it she asked if I read the label and I told her I had eaten it before. But after she left the room and I had eaten some of it, I decided to read the label and it had coconut oil in it! Mommy said for me to tell her immediately if I felt funny and she kept coming in and asking me how I felt. Mommy said the coconut oil in that popcorn must not have a nut protein in it so I was super lucky that time.

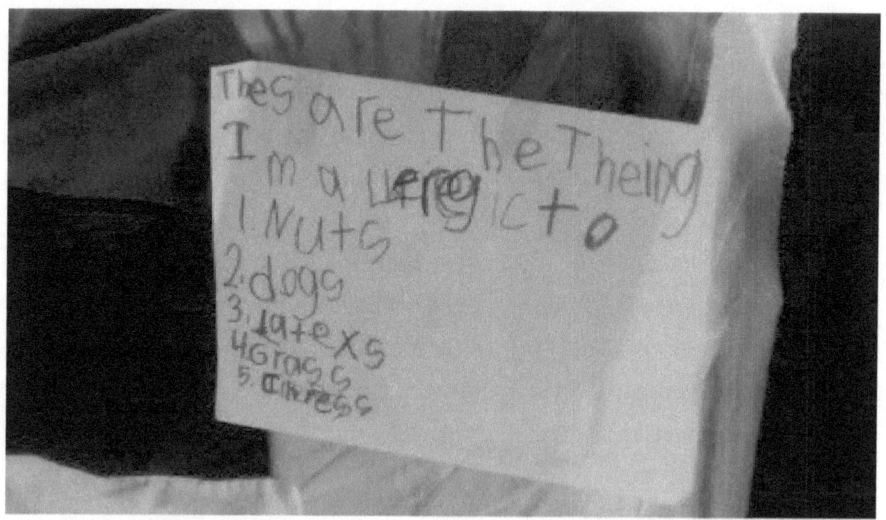

A sign Matthew made for his fort in 2016.

But is not just food. Nut oils are in everything. Coconut oil is in sunscreen and lip moisturizers. Almond oil is in shampoos, soaps and lotions. Matthew spent a week coughing day and night when we were on vacation. Once again, I thought he had a cold, but it sounded like his allergy cough. When we came home, I figured out the problem. My hair gel, that I used safely for over 10 years, had almond oil in it! I don't know if this was a new ingredient, or if this particular batch had a nut protein in it or if it was just because we were in a hotel room and so he was in close proximity to me when I was doing my hair, but he strongly reacted to it.

For us, there are no "safe" products. Ingredients change all the time, so we re-read the label every time we buy or use or eat anything. When we travel, I carry our own soaps, shampoos and lotions. We carry wet ones to wipe his hands if we aren't sure about the ingredients in the restroom soap. Matthew had a reaction at the dentist office when he had his teeth cleaned and we later learned the varnish they used was made with pine nuts. He had a reaction to some make-up I put on him for a play he was performing in – later I learned lots of eyeshadows and blushers are made with macadamia nut.

We were driving to the dress rehearsal of my play and my friend Claire was with us. I had put some make up on at Claire's house. And we were running late. All of a sudden I itched all over. Mommy told me to get the epi-pen bag and take out the wet ones and wipe off the make-up. I couldn't find it right away and I told Mommy I was scared. She pulled over in the church parking lot that has the skating rink and found the wipes and wiped off my face and hands and gave me some Benadryl. She told me if the itching didn't stop or get better in two minutes were going to have to go the hospital. Luckily it did. My friend Claire said, "now, we are really going to be late." I said "Claire, would you rather us be late or me be dead?!" Later on her mom told my mom Claire knew that was the wrong thing to say. Claire and I are still super good friends.

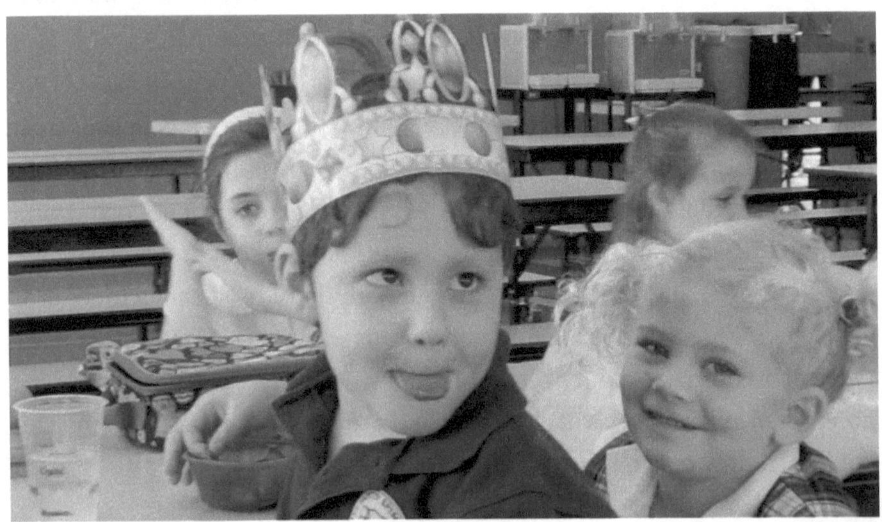

Matthew and Claire, 2016.

Matthew's allergy is so severe he can't be in the same room with people eating nuts. Kids eating Nutella (made with hazelnuts) at school in their classrooms and then playing with Matthew on the playground causes him to break out in hives. One time I ate a nut that accidentally fell on my salad while eating lunch in a restaurant. Thankfully, Matthew was not with me. But that night at dinner when I kissed him, he started coughing and hiving just from that contact I had with the nut six hours earlier. So, a nut free table at school does not ensure Matthew's safety. Only a nut free environment.

With allergies, the severity of the reaction intensifies every time you are exposed to it. Since Matthew is so allergic, we want to keep his exposure to an absolute minimum so that if he ever accidentally eats a tree nut or peanut, we have a better chance of the epi-pen working and saving his life. Something people with food allergies know and fear is that the epi-pen doesn't always prevent death. Sometimes the anaphylaxis is too quick and strong or the epi-pen is not administered quickly enough. This is the reality of Matthew's allergy and his life and it will probably never go away or get better.

I know someday I may have to inject myself with the epi-pen if I need it. And it scares me. I am afraid it will hurt like a shot.

4

Hardships, Blessings and Acts of Great Kindness.

Hard Stuff

When Matthew was four, we enrolled him in pre-K at a private school. My husband and I both attended private schools and really wanted Matthew to attend one as well. From the start Matthew did not like it. For my part, I was concerned they were not taking his allergy seriously enough. I told myself not to overreact and to give them a chance to implement a nut -free protocol. And I brushed aside Matthew's claims of dislike as just him taking time to adjust to a new environment. Things came to a crisis when I was at school assisting in the classroom in an effort to help him adjust. I saw that they made him sit separately from the other kids during meals and snacks, so he thought he was always in trouble. And they were letting kids bring anything they wanted in their lunches and snacks and all these kids shared a classroom, bathroom and playground. When I raised this issue with the principal – and I was admittedly upset at the time – she told me that maybe this school wasn't right for Matthew and we should look for another one. I was so shocked and angry I picked up Matthew and left without a word. An hour later we received an email telling us we had been dis-enrolled.

I hated that school. I don't remember much about the day we left. I have heard Mommy tell the story that she was crying. I remember we went back to my old pre-school and everyone was saying "hi" and was glad to see us. And I remember Mommy telling them we would be back tomorrow and I was so glad we were going back there.

I was so upset I cried all weekend – not because I wanted him at that school but because I had failed to protect my son and I ignored my instincts. At four, Matthew couldn't figure out that they were segregating him because of his allergy – he just thought he was in trouble and that no one liked to sit with him. He had loved school the previous year and had never been in trouble but now he was afraid every day that they would send him to time out. I felt horrible for putting him through this and I was so mad myself for not intervening the first minute I had a concern.

Never Again

After that, I vowed I would never "play nice" when it came to Matthew and his food allergies. Of course what that school did was illegal - food allergies are protected under the Americans with Disabilities Act - and as lawyers my husband and I knew that, but we do not want to force someone to care about Matthew's life. We decided we would chose a school that would care about keeping him safe and that was our highest criteria. And when it came to his safety I became proactive rather than reactive.

Every year, I send a letter to every parent in his class explaining his allergy. I speak about it in person again at the parent night. I meet with his teachers to explain the seriousness of his allergy and what keeping him safe entails. My husband and I have met with the head of the lower school and the head of the entire school on the rare occasions where we haven't felt his allergy was being handled properly. I communicate personally with every parent in Matthew's class if they forget and send a forbidden item. I keep snacks in the classroom for Matthew to have and share with others if somebody accidentally sends a food that he cannot be around. I have asked kids to throw away or put away food they have brought if it is harmful to Matthew and then I have bought them an alternate snack at the school snack bar. My husband or I go on every field trip and attend every party at the school. We go to every out of school party or play date. And everywhere Matthew goes we bring antihistamine and the epi-pen.

A Different Life

My friend Piper says some kids think I am lucky because they hate nuts and would be glad to be allergic. Or they don't believe I am allergic to every nut.

Matthew cannot attend day camps in the summer - we have literally been turned away at the door when they found out about his allergies and need for an epi-pen. Instead, he has spent every summer at home first with his Nanny and then with a trusted a babysitter. He only eats in a few "safe" restaurants and always the same items. He usually doesn't eat at parties or events for fear of cross contamination. And if he does eat, we almost always bring his own food. The vast majority of his playdates occur at our house as he can react just from being in a house where people eat a lot of nuts or have a nut tree on their property. We have never left him overnight- and he is 10 years old! He rarely goes to the grocery store. He has only been to one major league baseball game and that was before he developed the peanut allergy and never any other professional sports games. When we fly on an airplane, we wipe the entire seat, seat belt, arm rests and tray tables before Matthew sits down. We read the ingredients on every soap, lotion, make-up, sunscreen and food item before we use it or let Matthew use it. And everywhere Matthew goes we must carry the epi-pen and antihistamines. It is easy now as one of us just carries a backpack for him. But someday soon Matthew will have that responsibility and have to have ability to inject himself if needed. It is a scary prospect.

Blessings

Whenever I am explaining Matthew's allergies to people and the fact that he MUST be accommodated by them and their families, I say, "if it was not my kid, I would be totally annoyed having to do all this extra work!" And I am sympathetic to the inconvenience and the fact that people do forget about it sometimes. But after living with this every day for over 8 years and so far avoiding a life-threatening episode, I have come to see the blessings of it too.

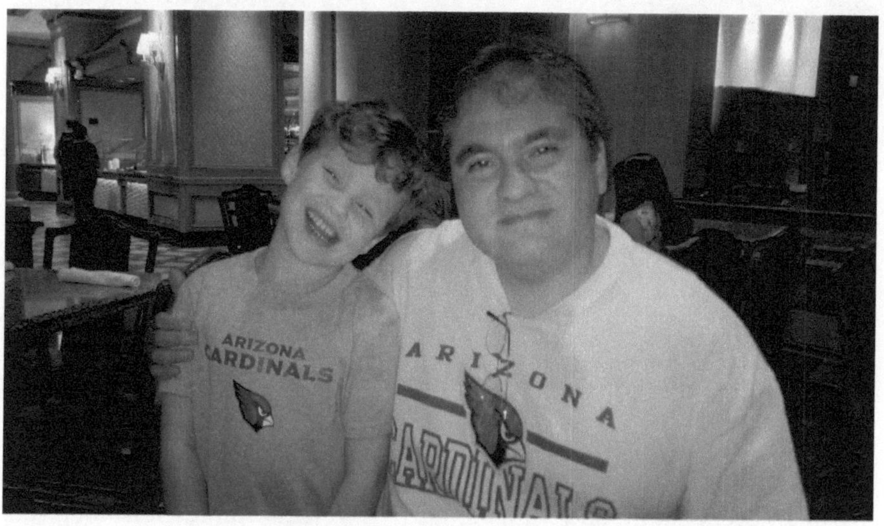

Matthew and Daddy, 2015

Matthew is always with us. My husband and I both spend considerably more time with him because of his allergy and have structured our lives around that. One of us picks him up every day and we rarely use weekend babysitters as there are few people we can trust to handle his allergy. For two people who work full-time as lawyers this has not always been easy, but it has been so worth it. Matthew is a naturally happy person, so he is a joy to be around and we call our nut-free threesome a "three-man party". I do not know that we would have given ourselves the permission to be this flexible and available to Matthew all the time if his allergy had not forced us.

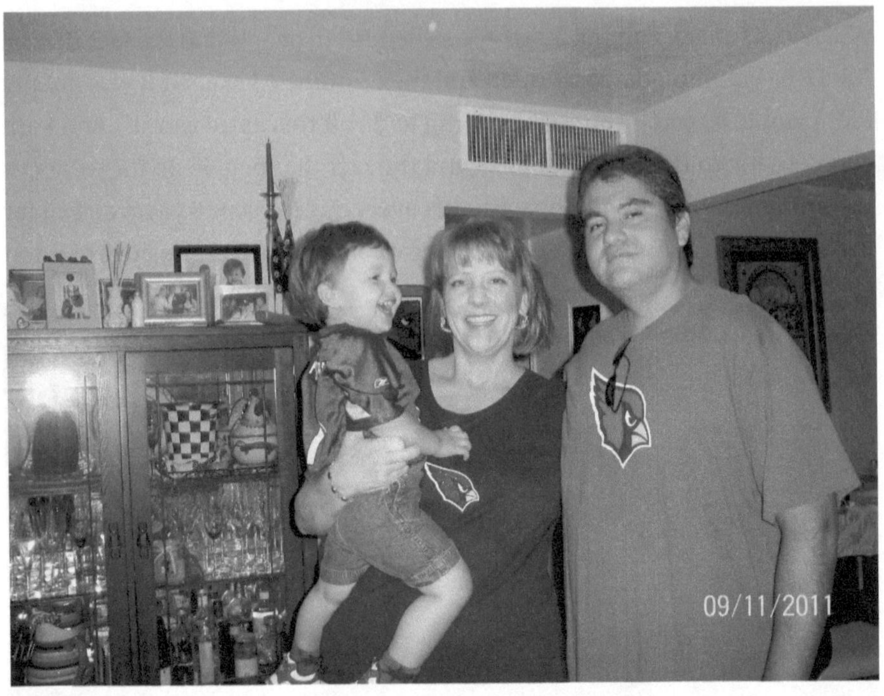

Three man party, 2011

We know every parent and child in Matthew's class. Granted it is not a very big school, but we are always there. I love being physically present, and the insight, knowledge, sense of community and accountability this gives us into Matthew's daily world. It is great to see all these relationships and influences on your child firsthand.

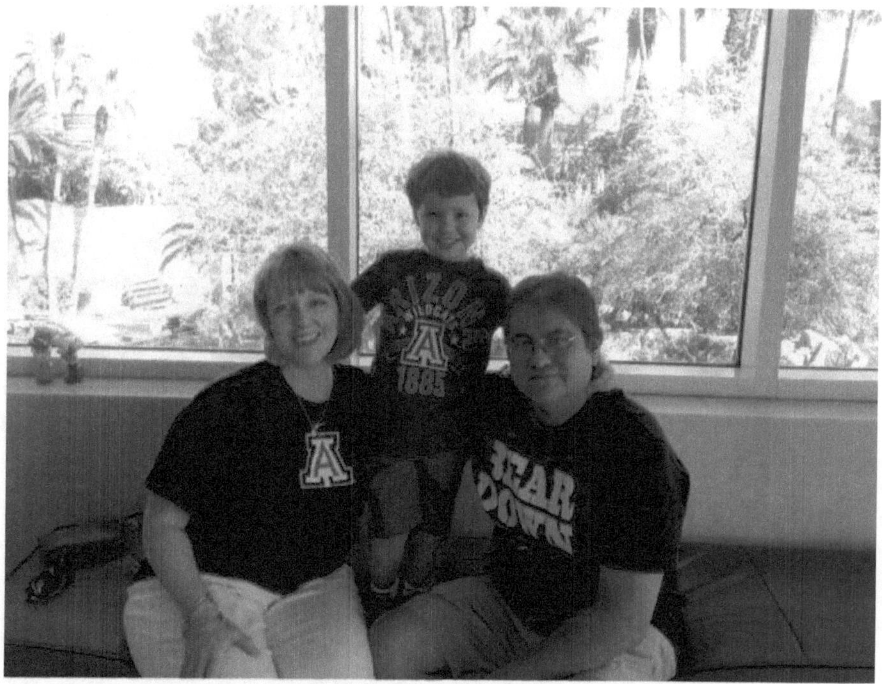

Three man party, 2015

Since it is hard to take Matthew to parties, we have a lot of parties at our house. We really get to spend quality time with our friends and his friends. We are the "go to" house for team parties and other get togethers. Matthew's birthday party guest list hovers between 75-100 people every year. All our friends and his friends and their families come. All these people are such a part of Matthew's life because he is always with us. It has given him a great sense of self and a huge loving supportive village.

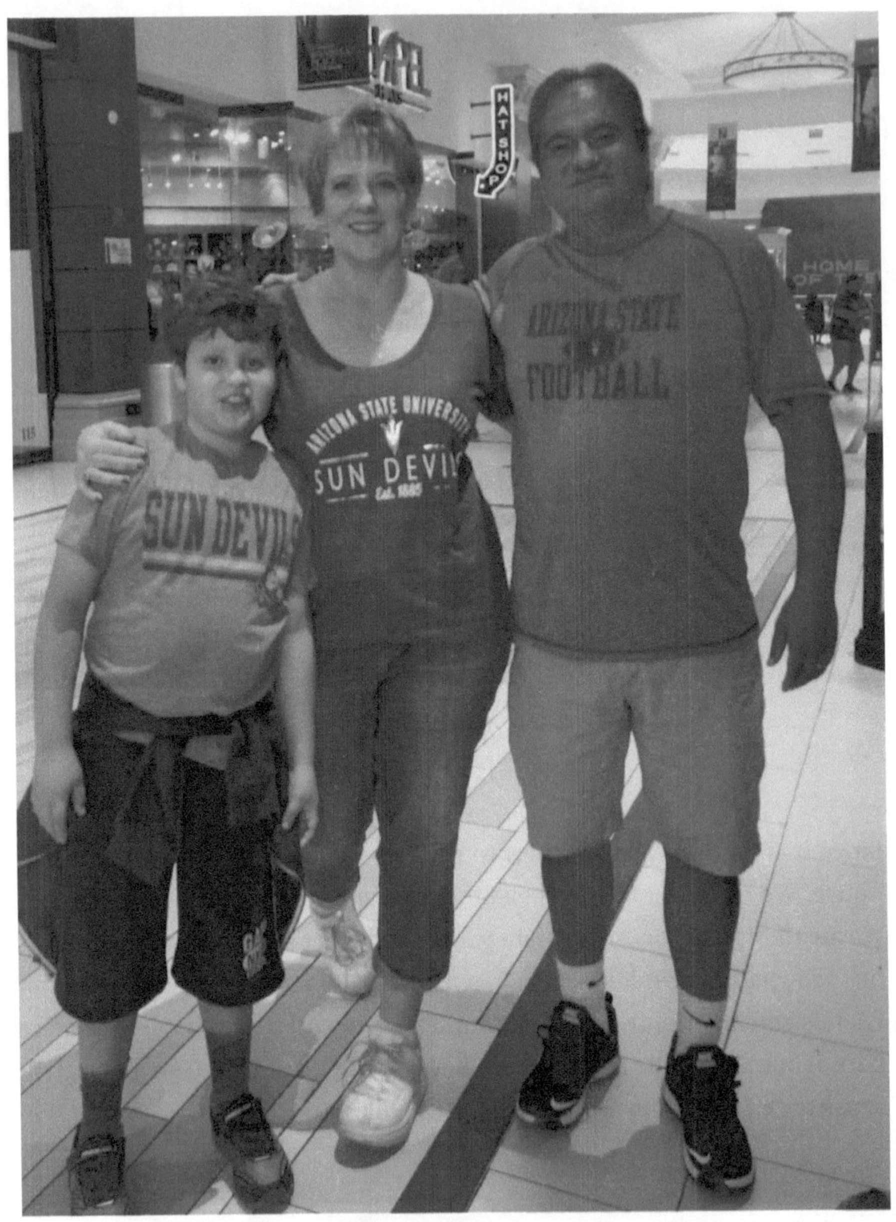

Three man party, 2018

Acts of Great Kindness

When I am with my friends they will ask me," Matthew, is this ok?" If I tell them it is not, they either throw it away or put it back in their lunch box. No one has ever been mean to me about my allergies. I mean why would they? I could die.

Over the years, we have seen acts of great kindness from people in response to Matthew's food allergies.

His godparents and their children always keep a nut free home and always refrain from eating nuts – just in case they see him.

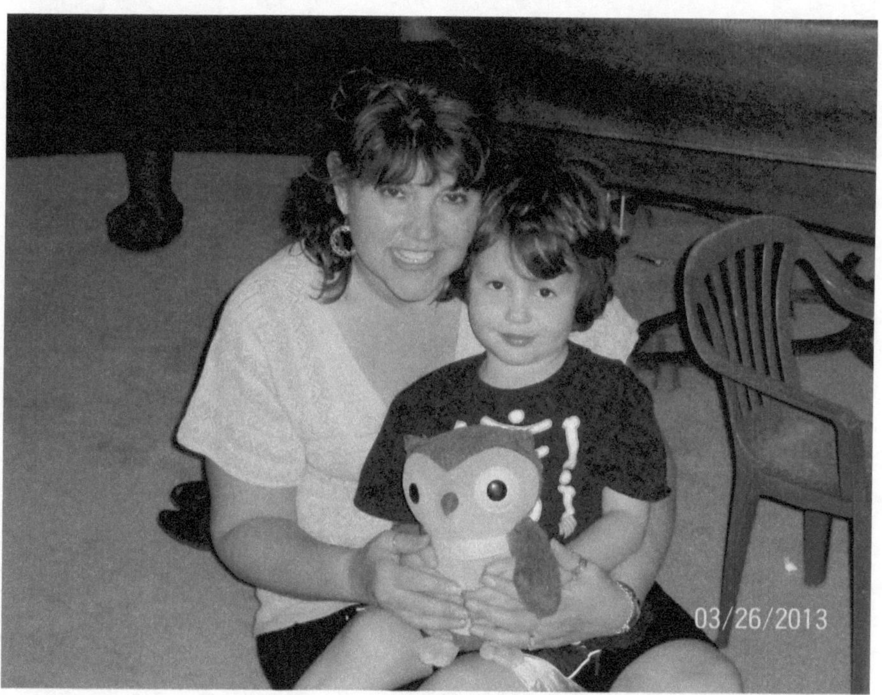

Matthew and his godmother, aka "Nina", Tracy in 2013

In kindergarten, his best friend Piper patrolled the lunch tables and told kids if they had to throw something away to keep Matthew safe. She still does it. We call her his "nut cop".

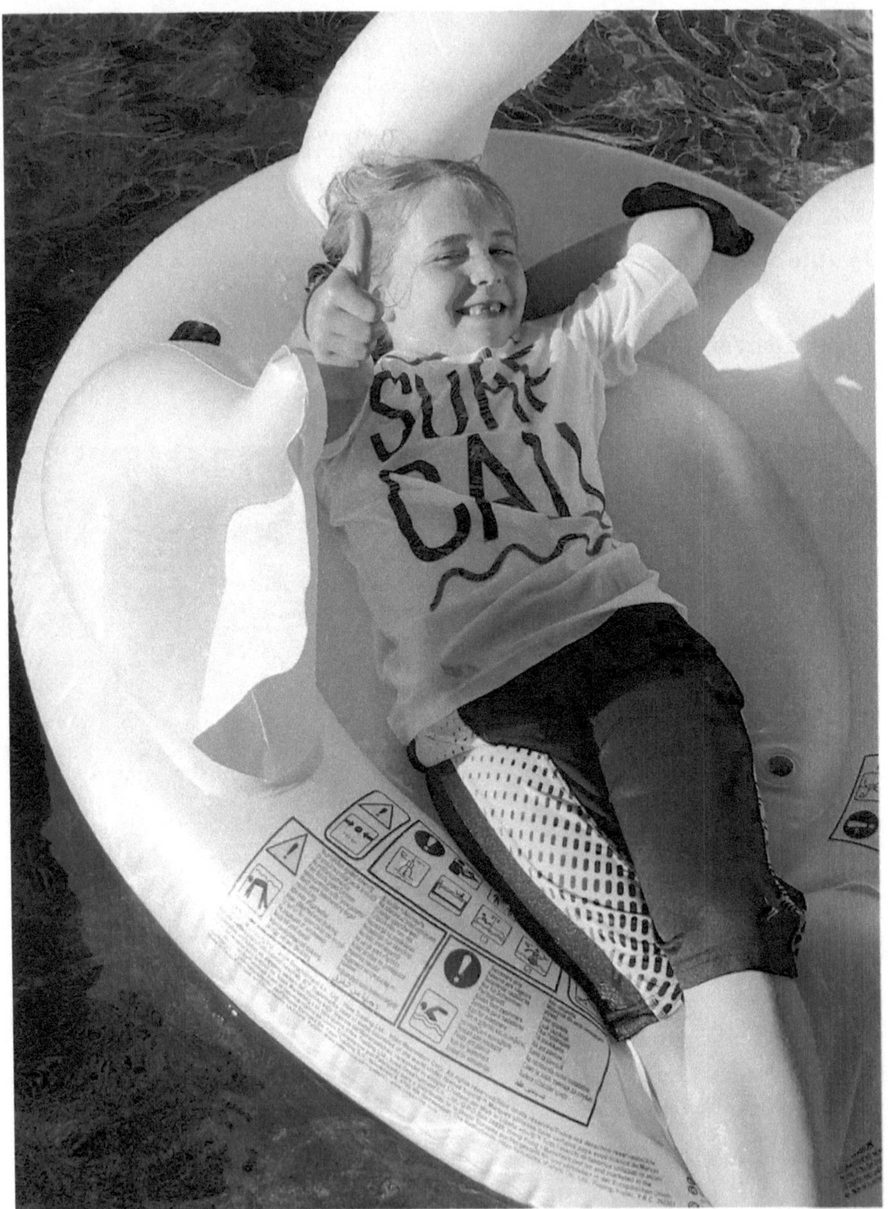

Piper, Matthew's "nut cop", 2018

His friend Justin told his mom that he did not want to bring a treat to share
with the class on his birthday unless it was something Matthew could and

would eat. There are lots of things that do not contain nuts but may be made in a facility that processes tree nuts. And Matthew doesn't like a lot of things and will not eat them because they have too many flavors - like cake. When that happens, he just eats some BBQ chips I have stored for him in his class room. But Justin was insistent that Matthew not be left out this time and brought chocolate donut holes for his treat - which are safe - and one of Matthew's favorites!

His friend Keaton will not ever eat peanut butter toast for breakfast "just in case Matthew wants to play with me today."

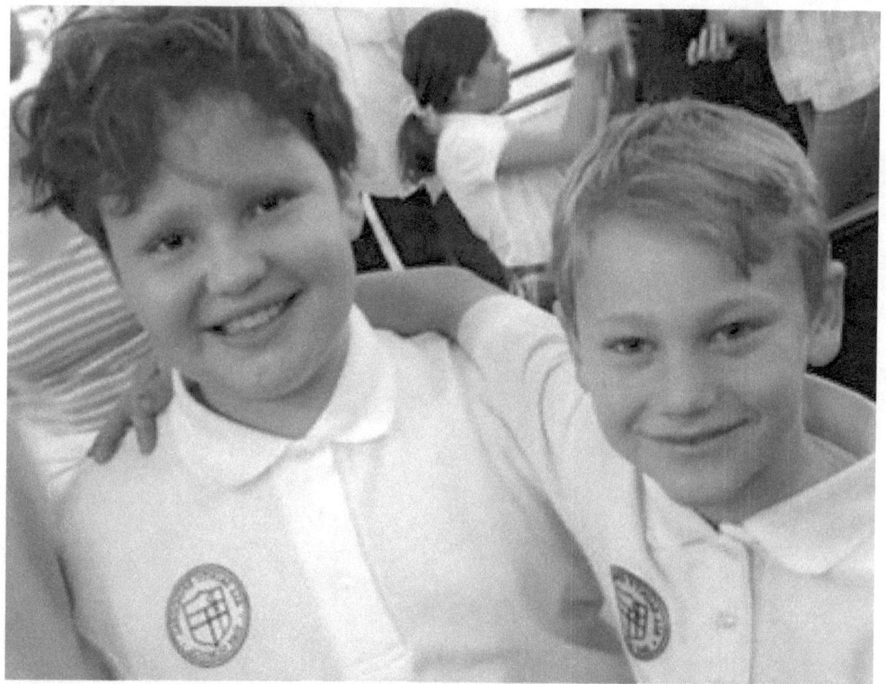

Matthew and Keaton, 2019

Charly and her older sister, Gabby, come over for all day long play dates in the summer. Matthew stays at home with his favorite babysitter Amanda because he cannot go to summer camps. These girls come and spend the day doing crafts, swimming and putting on plays at "Camp Amanda" with him. They have declined going to other camps and activities just to spend that time with him.

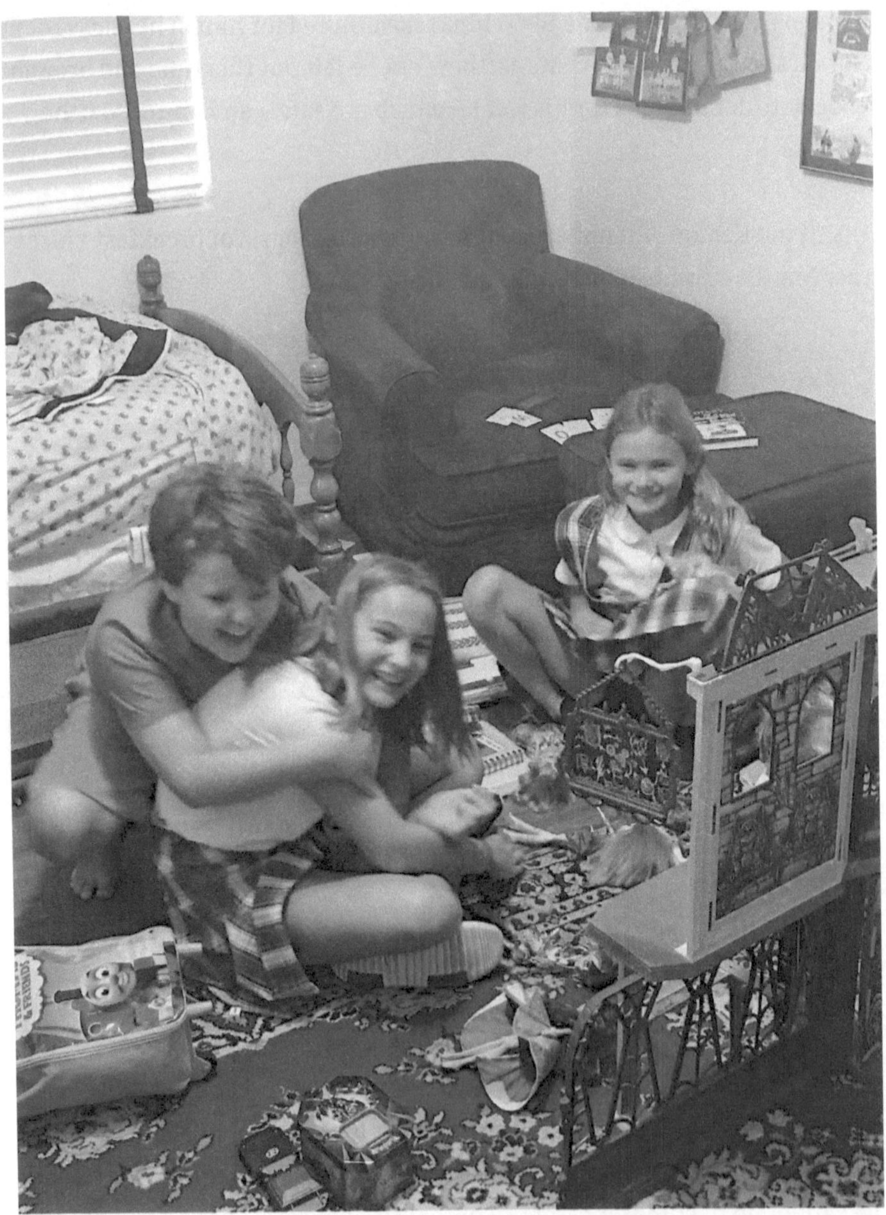

Matthew (hugging) Gabby and Charly, 2018

Abel, the school custodian, on his own initiative volunteered to heat up the corn tortilla quesadilla Matthew brings for lunch. They are homemade by his nanny for him and so very safe, healthy and his favorite food – but not as good when they are cold.

Kimberly's mom called to say she was bringing Rice Krispy treats for Kimberly's birthday and wanted to make sure Matthew could eat them. He can – but he doesn't like them. So, she brought him a KitKat instead.

His friend Claire, who was in the car with us when he had the serious reaction to make up, found out some kids were bringing nuts to school on purpose so they could sit together with their friends at a separate table instead of with their class. This third-grade girl requested a meeting with the teacher – on her own accord- and told him in no uncertain terms how dangerous this was for Matthew. I only learned about it after she had resolved it.

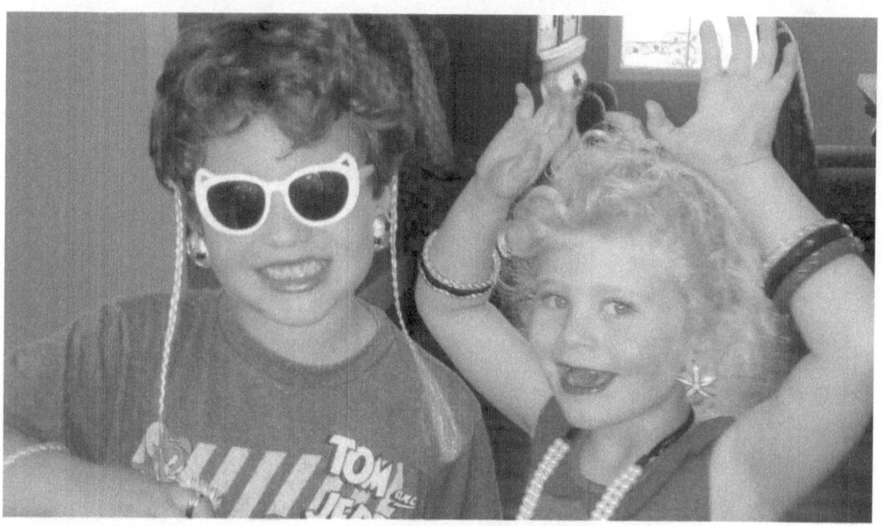

Matthew and Claire 2017, putting on a show

Max's mom was in charge of the second grade class project which was making dog treats to sell to raise money for animal shelters. She was having a hard time finding a recipe that did not contain peanut butter or coconut oil. Instead of excluding Matthew from the making of the treats part of the project and having him stay in the classroom with the teacher and work on tying the ribbons on the packages, she combined a few of the recipes together and had us come over to her house on a Sunday afternoon to test out which ones worked. Not only was it a fun play date for Matthew and Max, but we found a recipe that worked and Matthew got to participate in the fun part of class project.

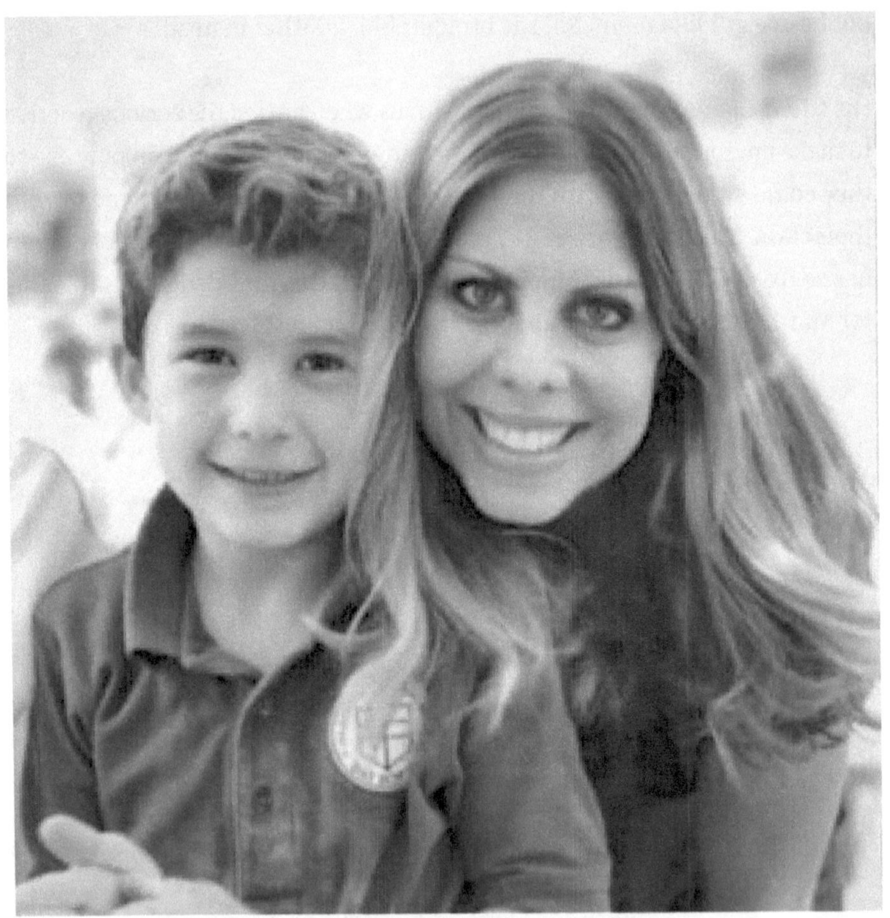

Max and his mom Katy, 2017

Piper and Will's parents bought a house very close to us. Piper and Will are twins who do not agree on much except their mutual love of Matthew. One of the first changes they made to this house was to remove a pecan tree from the back yard. They plan to make this house "nut free" so Matthew can come over anytime.

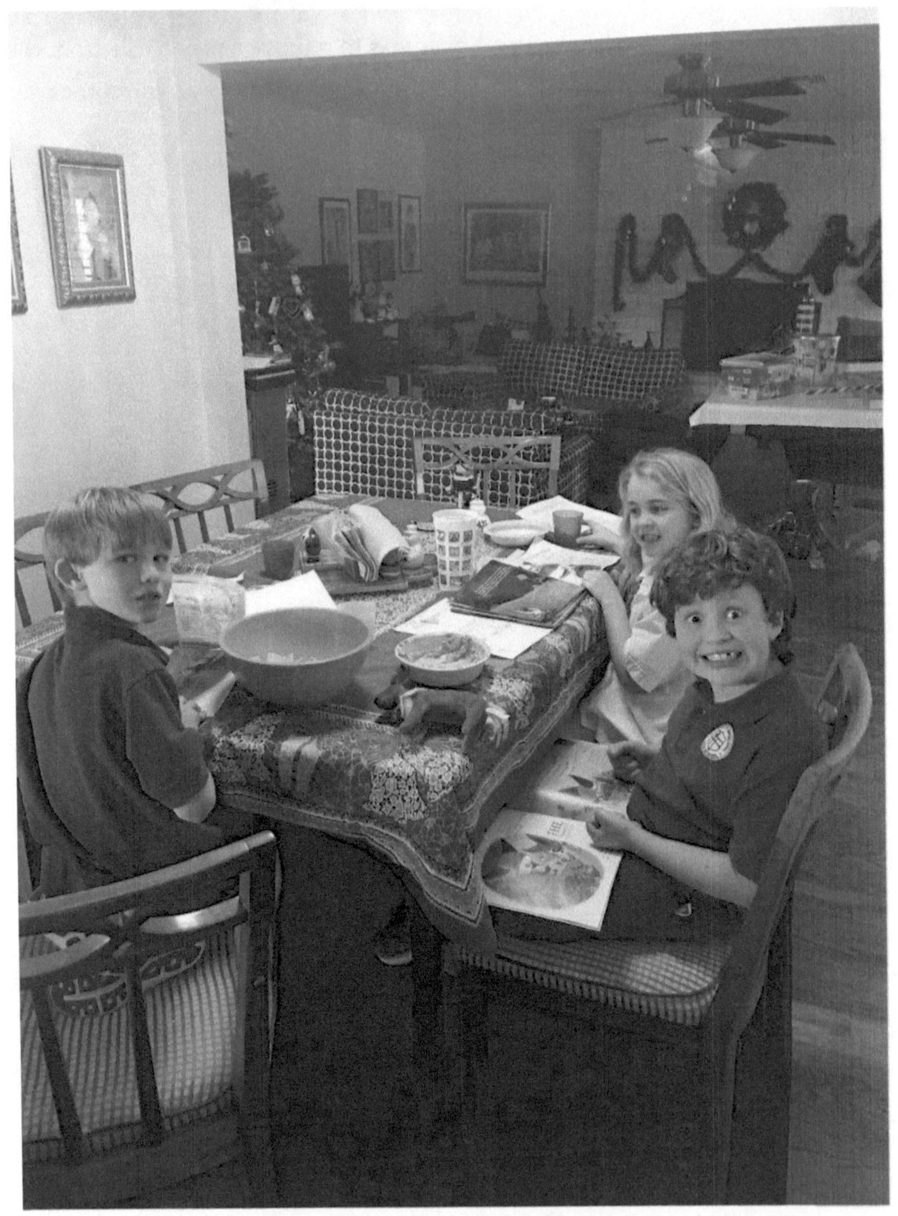

Matthew, Piper and Will, 2018

5

"So, What Now?"

People always ask if we think Matthew will outgrow his allergy. Hope springs eternal- but I seriously doubt it. Every year we have him re-tested. They do a blood test now. And every year his allergies are worse. For example, when they test for allergen specific IGE anti- bodies,3.50 – 17.4 kU/L is considered "high" and a class 3 allergy, meaning anaphylaxis is a concern. Matthew's IGE for walnuts is 53kU/L and a class 5 allergy! No wonder he had a reaction to that muffin all those years ago!

As Matthew gets older and his allergies worsen, some things are easier, and some things are harder. People don't touch him all the time like they did when he was a toddler. He can read ingredients. (And he doesn't need to get reading glasses first!) He is familiar with the symptoms and how it feels when he gets exposed to nuts. He has a talking "epi-pen" so it makes it easier for him to administer it to himself or for someone else to administer it. But I worry about bullying and push back from people for his accommodations. It would be easy to not include him in parties, activities or events and blame it on his food allergies.

So far, every child that has had to deal with his allergy has been amazing. But not every adult has. It enrages me when people act like his allergy is a "preference", and are inconvenienced when they have to accommodate him, and not the life-threatening condition that it is. I just have to pray that Matthew is able to confront people about this and stand up for himself when I am not there, so he stays safe and more importantly alive.

My friend Piper says my nut allergy makes me different but in a "good way". She says I am really brave and courageous because I am willing to go to places like airplanes and restaurants where they have nuts.

And there are experiences Matthew may never have and jobs he will probably never hold. He once listed his top five things he wanted to be when he grows up as 1) singer, 2) dancer, 3) actor, 4) elf and 5) baker. I had to tell him that with his nut allergy he would probably not be able to be a baker. And that if he wants to be a singer, dancer or actor he needs to get an accounting degree before going to acting school so he can support himself while waiting to get his big break or between gigs since he probably won't be able to wait tables like many other artists do. (I actually put that in the blessings column!) I don't think his allergy will affect him being an elf – so that remains an option.

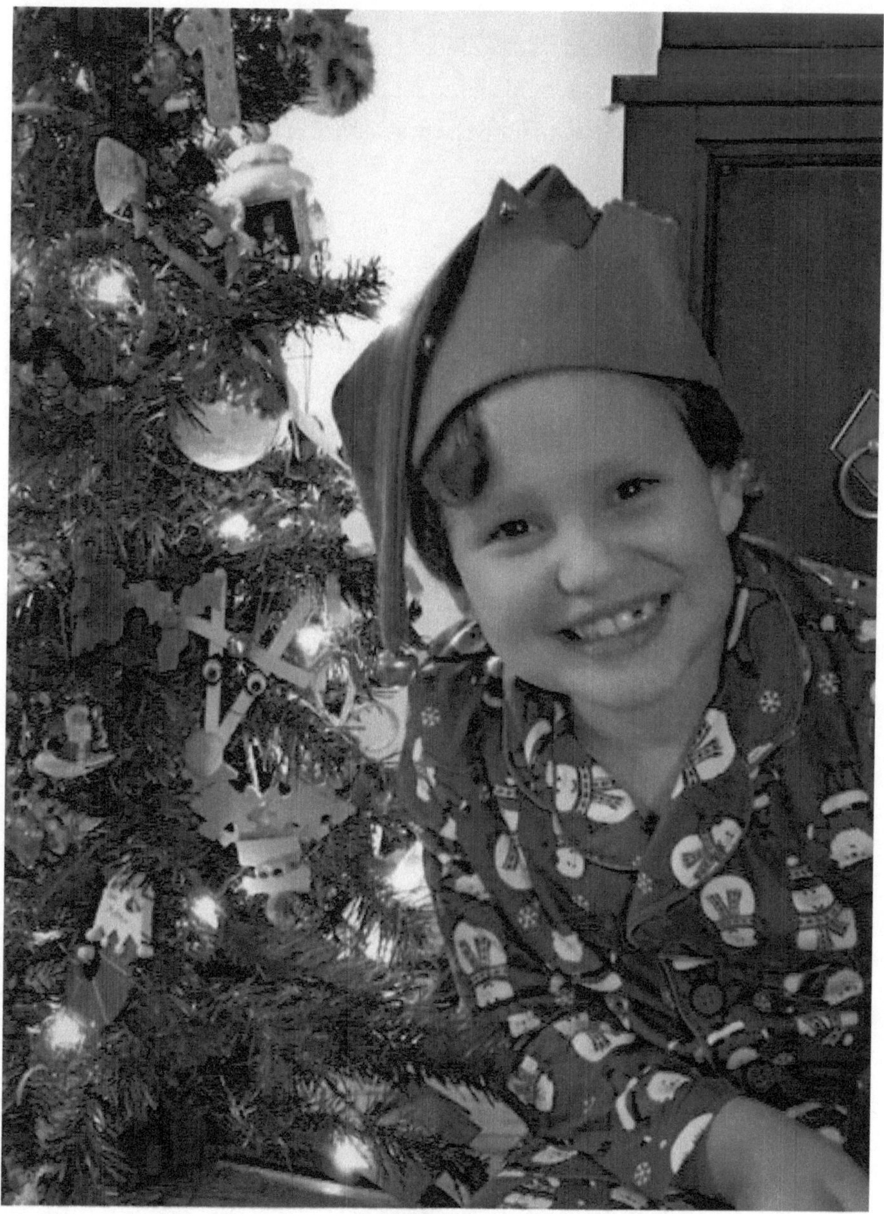

Matthew the elf

I don't know how much Matthew will ever be able to travel, especially overseas. Nuts are prevalent in the foods of many cultures and the language barriers combined with a lack of understanding of food allergies, as they are very rare in other countries, I fear it would be too much of a risk. I am not even sure he will ever be able to go to Hawaii with the prevalence of coconut and macadamia nut foods!

Matthew's social encounters may be different too. He may not ever be a guy you meet for "lunch" – unless you want to meet at the two restaurants he can go to. Food is a different experience for him and not particularly social. So much food is forbidden to him that he sticks with a pretty limited menu. But as I mentioned before, since he has been around them his whole life, he will probably throw one heck of a party!

I live a normal life except when it comes to food. If I gave advice to someone with my allergies I would say check every label and chose wisely what you eat. But keep calm because you might grow out of it. And try to make the most of your life.

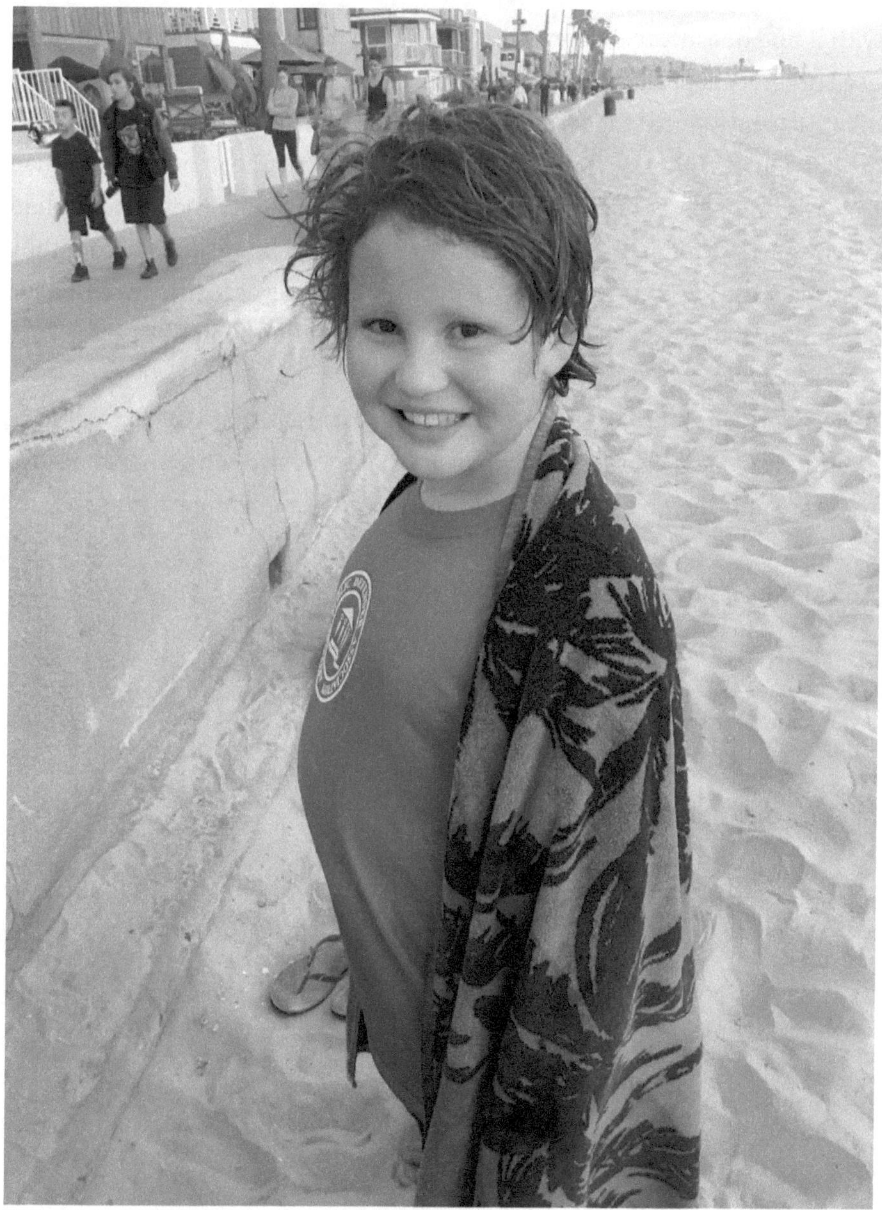

Matthew , 2018

The best thing of all about Matthew and this journey is that he is totally fine with it and doesn't feel deprived at all. When he was in kindergarten, they used to serve fudgesicles at the school snack bar that were made with coconut oil. (They have since stopped.) One day, all his friends were eating them after school and playing tag. Not only could Matthew not have one, but we had to leave immediately because he couldn't be touched by the kids that had eaten them. (Kindergarten boys and tag? It would be seconds before they were all wrestling on the ground like puppies!) Whenever Matthew can't have something that is served or offered, we always get him something else.

As we were on our way to get him a different treat that day I asked him, "Matthew, do you ever feel bad when you have to leave somewhere because there are nuts or you can't eat something because it might have nuts?"

And Matthew said, "*No, that is just the way God made me.*"

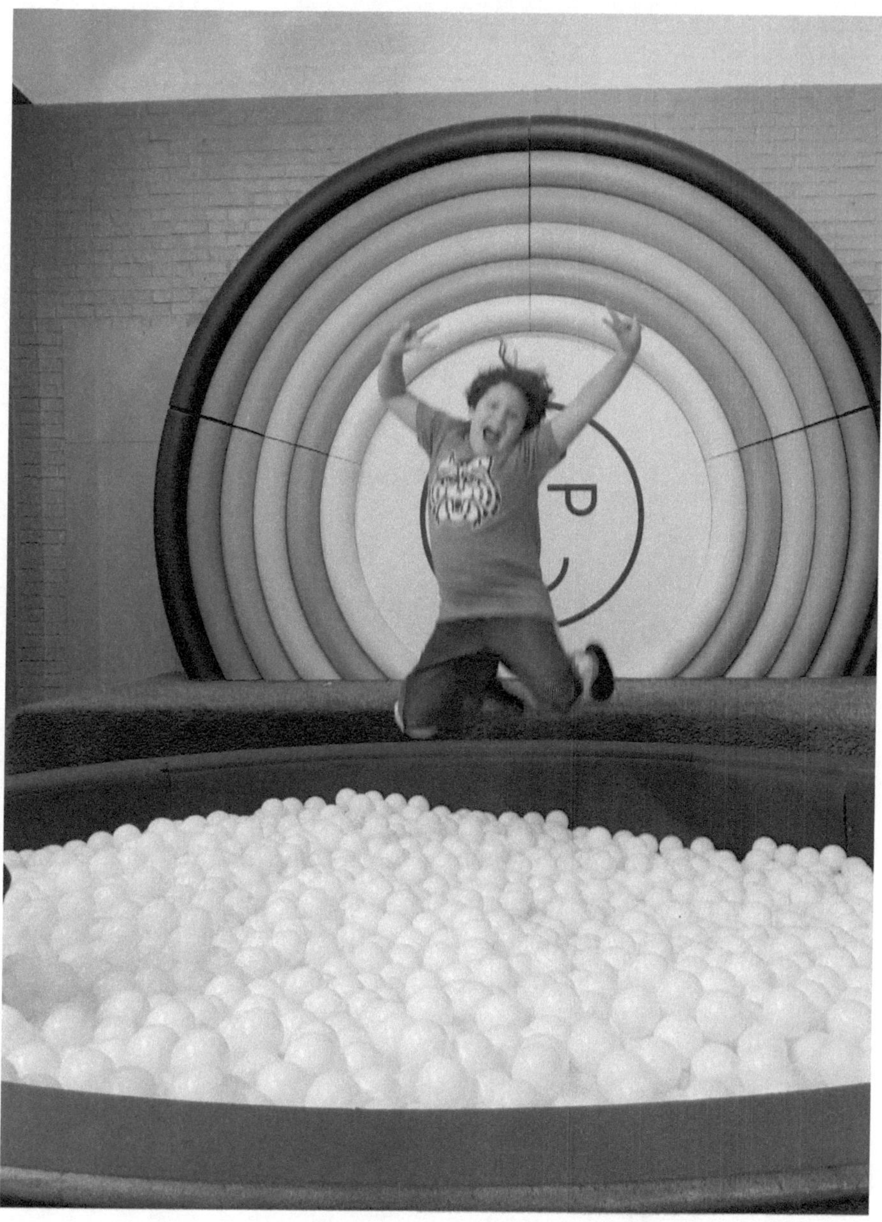

Matthew, 2019

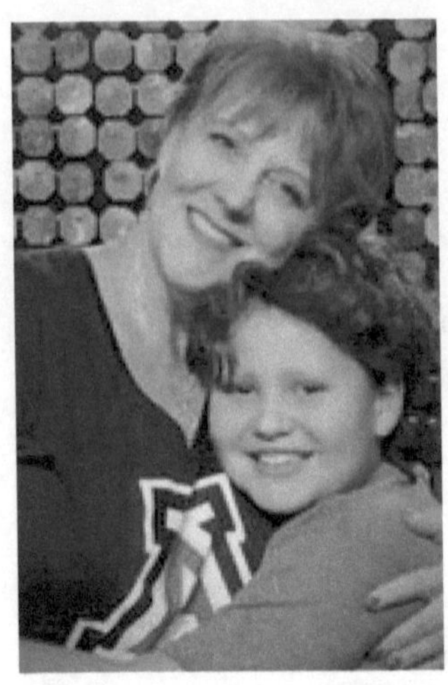

About the Author

Meg and Matthew Leal live in Phoenix, Arizona with Daddy and Murray Cat. This is their second book. Thank you to everyone in Matthew's life who share this journey with him and shower him and us with their kindness and understanding and for letting us use their stories and pictures. Matthew always says he is a very lucky person and he is right!

www.ingramcontent.com/pod-product-compliance
Lightning Source LLC
Chambersburg PA
CBHW051424250726
48655CB00003B/1218